THE LONGEVITY PARADOX

HOW TO DIE YOUNG AT A RIPE OLD AGE

BY STEVEN R. GUNDRY

Mercy Brain

Disclaimer

This book is a summary and meant to be a great companionship to the original book or to simply help you get the gist of the original book.

Table of Contents

1 Minute Overview

From the creator of the New York Times smash hit The Plant Paradox comes a historic arrangement for carrying on with a long, sound, cheerful life.

From the minute we are conceived, our cells start to age. Be that as it may, maturing does not need to mean decrease. Incredibly famous specialist Dr. Steven Gundry has been treating developed patients for the greater part of his profession. He realizes that everybody supposes they need to live perpetually until they hit middle age and witness the enduring of their folks and even their companions. So how would we settle the mystery of needing to live to a ready maturity—however, appreciate the advantages of youth?

This notable book holds the appropriate response. Working with a huge number of patients, Dr. Gundry has found that the "maladies of maturing" we most dread is not just an element of age; rather, they are a side-effect of the manner in which we have lived throughout the decades. In the Longevity Paradox, he maps out another way to deal with maturing admirably—one that depends on supporting the soundness of the "most established" portions of us: the microorganisms that live inside our bodies.

Our gut bugs—the microorganisms that make up the microbiome—to a great extent decide our wellbeing throughout the years. From infections like disease and Alzheimer's to regular illnesses like joint inflammation to our weight and the presence of our skin, these bugs are in the driver's seat, controlling our personal satisfaction as we age.

The uplifting news is, it's never past the point where it is possible to help these organisms and give them what they must support them—and you—flourish. In the Longevity Paradox, Dr. Gundry traces nourishment and way of life intended to help gut wellbeing and live well for quite a long time to come. A dynamic interpretation of the new investigation of maturing, The Longevity Paradox offers an activity intend to counteract and turn around sickness just as basic hacks to enable anybody to look and feel more youthful and progressively indispensable.

INTRODUCTION: THIS IS A TEST

As a heart specialist, I have done my part to broaden the lives of many people. I'm pleased with the way that I've helped such a large number of individuals live longer lives, however I quit my place of employment as teacher and head of cardiothoracic medical procedure at Loma Linda University School of Medicine when I discovered that much of what I'd been educated about wellbeing and life span— data that numerous driving specialists still accept is valid— was just off-base.

For as long as nineteen years, I've been treating my patients with a blend of nourishing treatment and ordinary prescription, and again and again, I've seen unbelievable outcomes. At the point when my patients treat their gut amigos right, they can drastically increment their life expectancies. As my patients and regular readers know, I've seen sensational inversions of sicknesses that numerous specialists still accept are irreversible, changes that we can follow refined blood work and that my patients can feel and see. A significant number of these progressions are straightforwardly connected to adjustments we've made to their gut microbes.

Between the outcomes I've seen in my patients, my investigation of a gigantic measure of late research on the gut biome, and my own investigations of the world's longest-lived networks, I currently realize that your gut microorganisms as it was impacting both to what extent you'll live and how well you'll live. Furthermore, with the assistance of my astounding patients, I've assembled a program that will drive out the terrible folks and make the heroes feel protected and cheerful in their home, so they'll be constrained to totally revive their neighborhood both all around.

A few components of the Longevity Paradox program might be recognizable, for example, eating loads of specific vegetables and getting the correct measures of activity and rest, while others, for example, deceiving your body into believing it's winter year round to invigorate your foundational microorganisms and dispersing out your dinners to "wash" your cerebrum around evening time, are fresh out of the box new. These techniques have helped my patients lower their circulatory strain and cholesterol markers, essentially diminish manifestations of joint inflammation and other joint issues, resolve MS, lupus, and other immune system conditions, improve heart wellbeing, and moderate or switch the movement of disease what's more, dementia—also shed pounds and look decades more youthful! What's more, they achieve this without starving, eating twigs, checking calories, or putting in hours at the exercise center.

It doesn't make a difference how old you are, the means by which old you feel, or how debilitated or sound you might be at the present time. As on most of the best home-makeover appears, remodels happen immediately when the general population in control have the correct materials and are roused to take care of business. On the off chance that you pursue my arrangement, inside only half a month you'll have more gut pals and far fewer squatters, and you'll begin to see and feel a distinction in your vitality levels, in your absence of side effects of a considerable lot of the most regular infections of maturing, on your skin, and on the scale.

So how about we begin changing your body into the most alluring oceanfront suite available for your gut microorganisms. They'll make sure to thank you with a long and solid life.

Key Takeaway:
- What you eat matters
- Research shows that you can control your health with your food
- Not all medications are helpful

I: The Aging Myths

Before we get into precisely how to best deal with your gut amigos, how about we take a more critical take a gander at how they work in your body and for what reason they're such a basic part of your wellbeing and life span. While we're grinding away, we'll clear up a few disarray, deception, and out and out lies about how and why we age.

With regards to your gut microscopic organisms, you have two needs. To start with, you have to make the great ones so upbeat that they'll need to stick around and keep their home beautiful and very much thought about and influence the terrible ones so troubled that they'll escape the premises for good. This will give you the perfect populace and decent variety of gut pals that you requirement for a long life expectancy and wellbeing range. Second, it's simply as fundamental to have a solid gut lining, which I and different specialists allude to as the fringe or mucosal boundary, to keep those gut mates where they ought to be (in your intestinal tract) so they can shield you from outside intruders and stay away from being confused with intruders themselves. A solid, impermeable boundary is the key to maintaining a strategic distance from huge numbers of the maladies we partner with "ordinary" maturing.

How about we begin with your gut microscopic organisms: what they are, their main thing, and why they are such a critical bit of the Longevity Paradox.

CHAPTER 1: ANCIENT GENES CONTROL YOUR FATE

I have seen numerous patients who are lacking in a few nutrients, minerals, and proteins when they come to me—not on the grounds that they aren't expending them but since their microbiome isn't fabricating or potentially permitting retention of them. When we drive out the awful bugs and propel these patients' gut pals to rejuvenate the area, lo and see, the inadequacies vanish. You can consider it along these lines: you are not what you eat; you are what your gut mates digest. What's more, they can process just the nourishment they have advanced to perceive and process for you.

To include a note of levity here, one of the best extensive wellbeing masters of the twentieth century, Jack LaLanne, whom I had the joy of knowing, used to give this exhortation on eating: "In the event that it tastes great, spit it out!" What he was really saying without knowing it at the time was: eat for them, not for you! Furthermore, cheer up; the sustenance you will eat for them will taste extraordinary for you, I guarantee.

In any case, your gut mates have a lot of different occupations, as well. They keep yeast, or candida (which is a typical occupant of each gut), in line and battle against the excess of other hurtful microorganisms. They additionally go about as bouncers, keeping an eye on the way to your gut and really teaching your invulnerable framework as to which nourishments and substances are advantageous (or best case scenario innocuous) and ought to be let in and which ones may hurt you and ought to be banished from the section. This specific occupation has turned out to be progressively requesting throughout the years as our weight control plans have turned out to be progressively unpredictable (more on this later).

Your gut amigos likewise make the forerunners to numerous essential hormones and speak with the remainder of the cells in your body about how life is going down in the gut. How precisely do they do this? In addition to other things, by flagging specifically to your mitochondria, obviously! Did you ponder those very astute old dealmakers that jumped into our cells for a superior spot to live what's more, security and in return do the critical activity of creating the majority of the vitality we requirement for our cells? Obviously not. Actually, I trust they speak to a missing connection in many discourses about life span.

You acquired both your gut amigos and your mitochondria from your mom. As a boost, mitochondria are overwhelmed microbes that live in the entirety of your cells. They contain their own mitochondrial DNA (qualities) that really isolate independently from the remainder of the cell's DNA contained in the core. All mitochondrial DNA is transmitted through the female egg from mother to baby. So all mitochondria and their DNA are female. In like manner, your mom at first populated your gut microbiome during childbirth with her microorganisms as you went down the birth trench and were presented to the microorganisms in her vagina.

This exquisite framework proceeded much further when your mom breastfed you for the first run through. Incredibly, her milk contained explicit sugar particles called oligosaccharides and galactooligosaccharides that you couldn't process however were the definite kind of sustenance the gut amigos she'd quite recently passed onto you preferred best. In different words, Mom was nourishing two newborn children on the double: you and your recently presented (from her) microbiome. She expected to get you two off to an extraordinary beginning—a reality that is mind-blowing as well as, as you'll before long learn, personality advancing!

In this manner, I like to think about your gut amigos and your mitochondria, which both originated from your mom, as sisters. What's more, similar to all the best sisters, they are continually conversing with one another. (In any event that is the situation with my own two little girls.) Your gut pals answer to their sister mitochondria about what's occurring in their edge of the townhouse, and the mitochondria react to those reports by taking one of a few activities. Notwithstanding making vitality for your cells, mitochondria are responsible for cell flagging, cell separation (what sort of cell a given cell ought to move toward becoming), cell passing, and cell development. In other words, the mitochondria choose if a cell ought to develop quickly, gradually, or not at all. We will see this again later when we talk about malignant growth cells.

Take Away
- Your gut microbes have been with you since birth
- Your gut determines your overall health
- There is a correlation between cancer and gut health

CHAPTER 2: PROTECT AND DEFEND

Having the correct gut pals in your microbiome is just 50% of the condition. The second half is ensuring they remain on their side of the intestinal fringe. At the point when bits of their phone dividers called lipopolysaccharides (LPSs, which we will speak increasingly about in a moment) cross the fringe from your gut to your organs, tissues, lymph, or blood, it doesn't make a difference if they're gut mates or awful bugs. Any microscopic organisms, LPSs, or different trespassers sneaking where they don't have a place trigger a resistant reaction that produces across the board aggravation and lays the basis for quickened maturing and ailment.

Your stomach acids, chemicals, and gut pals separate the sustenance you eat into individual parts: amino acids (from protein), unsaturated fats (from fat), also, sugar particles (from sugars and starches). Your mucosal cells then actually gnaw off a solitary atom of these processed amino acids, unsaturated fats, and sugars, go it through the body of the cell, and discharge it into your entry vein or lymph framework. At the point when all is functioning admirably, everything other than these single particles stays outside the intestinal obstruction, where it has a place. There is a great deal of truth to

Robert Frost's lyric that says, "Great wall make great neighbors." If your mucosal cells are arranged firmly one next to the other, your gut lining capacities as a "great fence" that keeps everything with the exception of single atoms of processed amino acids, unsaturated fats, and sugar on the opposite side. Be that as it may, if your fence gets worn out, what's more, ends up overflowing with minuscule gaps, it will enable different mixes to spill through, and your wellbeing will start to endure. This is the meaning of "flawed gut," otherwise called intestinal penetrability, and it is at the heart (or will I say gut?) of the vast majority of the normal infections we partner with maturing. Indeed, as you will before long observe, it's the steady breakdown of this obstruction that quickens the maturing process.

That is on the grounds that when the wrong particles or even microscopic organisms cross the outskirt, the safe framework kicks into high apparatus. It's useful to think about the resistant framework as the police power of your inner apartment suite. When they discover that somebody has broken in, the cops flood the scene and call for fortifications by discharging fiery hormones called cytokines. It's incredible to have these "cops" around when you truly need them. For instance, if the "miscreant" that breaks your intestinal coating is really unsafe, for example, a bacterial contamination, they can spare your life. When you have damage, aggravation can enable you to recuperate. Be that as it may issues happen when the cops get brought again and again for each easily overlooked detail. The result is incessant irritation, a definitive reason for the regular maladies of maturing, from Alzheimer's to malignancy, diabetes, and immune system illnesses.

Take Away:
- Sugar feeds the cells you need to starve
- Microbes in your gut protect your body
- The wrong foods irritate your gut and cause you to have problems

CHAPTER 3: WHAT YOU THINK IS KEEPING YOU YOUNG IS PROBABLY MAKING YOU OLD

Numerous alleged wellbeing masters take a gander at the rundown of Blue Zones and, seeing that two of the longest-living societies are found on islands in the Mediterranean, exhort their devotees to just pursue the Mediterranean eating routine, which incorporates grains.

However, a more critical take a gander at those societies uncovers that oat grains are really a negative part of the Mediterranean eating regimen, implying that these people live long, solid lives in spite of eating such huge numbers of grains, not as a result of it. Actually, due to their dependence on grains, Italians by and large have fundamentally high rates of joint inflammation, and Sardinians specifically have a high extent of immune system ailments.

Our gut pals, even in these enduring networks, still haven't adjusted to eating grains, and that incorporates the new "in" grains, for example, quinoa furthermore, farro. The same number of my Peruvian patients let me know, their moms instructed them continuously to weight cook quinoa to evacuate the poisons; and farro is simply wheat, plain and basic, however with a gussied-up name.

Creature protein was before the rarest and most costly kind of nourishment and still is in the vast majority of the Blue Zones. In any case, in the West, it has moved toward becoming ludicrously cheap gratitude to government sponsorships of the corn, different grains, and soybeans that are encouraged to modernly cultivated creatures, poultry, and even fish. The result is that numerous Western social orders boundlessly overconsume creature protein, driving to higher glucose levels, heftiness, and a shorter life expectancy.

Still not persuaded that you should restrict your utilization of creature protein? Try not to stress; it took me some time to arrive, as well. As a kid from Nebraska, I grew up eating loads of "sound" red meat. Yet, my time at Loma Linda College showed me generally. My previous partner at Loma Linda Dr. Gary Fraser has directed an investigation of the seemingly perpetual Seventh-Day Adventists and run a meta-investigation of six different examinations.

His outcomes plainly demonstrate that veggie lover SeventhDay Adventists who eat no creature items live the longest, trailed by veggie lover Seventh-Day Adventists who eat restricted measures of eggs and no dairy items. Vegan Seventh-Day Adventists who devour dairy items come straightaway, and Seventh-Day Adventists who once in a while eat chicken or fish raise the back as far as life span.

Unfortunately, creature protein is basically not an important element for a long wellbeing range. As Dr. Fraser has illustrated, totally keeping away from creature protein delivered the best life span among an as of now incredibly extensive individuals. Further, the danger of building up Alzheimer's ailment connects specifically with the measure of meat devoured.

The numbers don't lie. Investigations of US war veterans, expired proficient baseball players, and French people (an odd gathering of people, however bear with me) all demonstrate an opposite connection among tallness and life span.

Many examines additionally uncover an association among tallness and malignancy. In one investigation, fast development amid immaturity brought about a 80 percent expanded danger of disease after fifteen years.

Stop at the present time and read that measurement once more—a 80 percent expanded danger of malignant growth! Need another chilling certainty? When I was in therapeutic school during the 1970s, youngsters' malignant growth wards contained just a bunch of beds; presently they possess entire towers or even whole emergency clinics.

My associates directing another examination partitioned in excess of 22,000 solid male specialists in the United States into five classifications dependent on stature and caught up with them twelve years after the fact. Indeed, even in the wake of modifying for the specialists' ages, the outcomes showed a positive relationship among tallness and the improvement of malignant growth.

This is startling, however it bodes well since high IGF-1 levels, brought about by mTOR detecting vitality in the body, advances cell development. This incorporates development of both the cells that assistance us develop tall and the cells that become malignant. contemplates on people demonstrate that having expanded iron in the blood as a individual ages expands his or her danger of building up Alzheimer's ailment. And in those without Alzheimer's, mind imaging innovation has uncovered a predictable connection between's subjective brokenness and iron statement.

There is even a recently perceived type of cell demise called ferroptosis that is connected to something over the top iron in the cerebrum! Yet another examination on the impacts of iron on mind work demonstrated that when Parkinson's patients diminished their iron dimensions by giving blood, their indications were significantly diminished.

Iron is fantastically maturing, and it's found in a colossal supply, obviously, in creature protein So how about we take a gander at a portion of the fat sources that are best for life span. Not fortuitously, they all originate from plants. What's more, Dr. Keys, who was no sham, picked olives and olive oil. Olive oil's principle fat is a monounsaturated fat, oleic corrosive, yet it's not this fat secures against coronary illness, subjective decrease, Alzheimer's malady, and neurological aggravation. It's in reality all the polyphenols that are contained in olive oil that have the effect.

This is fundamentally in light of the fact that these plant mixes invigorate autophagy, your cells' reusing program. Remember what sends the flag to your cells to animate autophagy—your gut pals, obviously. Our gut amigos love the polyphenols in olive oil, and I endeavor to devour a liter of it seven days, as individuals in a considerable lot of the Blue Zones do. Nuts are additionally uncommonly high in monounsaturated and polyunsaturated fat and are astoundingly defensive against coronary illness. Why? Since they, and the prebiotic fiber they contain, are additionally cherished by your gut pals! Eating pistachios, walnuts, and almonds (stripped, it would be ideal if you expands your dimension of butyrate-creating microscopic organisms, with walnuts and pistachios beating almonds in a avalanche. A portion of my companions in the paleo network are additionally amped up for the astounding impacts of butyrate and attempt to get a greater amount of it by eating extra spread (fun truth: butyrate is named after margarine). Spread is surely a modest wellspring of butyrate, at the same time, tragically, it's anything but a smart thought to eat a ton of dairy items on the off chance that you need to carry on with a long and sound life. Also, that drives me to our seventh and last legend. Amid assimilation, casein A1 can transform into beta-casomorphin-7, a narcotic peptide that joins to the pancreas' insulin-delivering cells and prompts an insusceptible assault (and subsequently aggravation). This is likely an essential reason for sort 1 diabetes.

The most well-known type of dairy animals worldwide is the Holstein, whose milk contains this tricky protein. Numerous individuals see that milk gives them gastrointestinal issues or makes them overproduce bodily fluid, which as you most likely are aware at this point is one of our body's real barrier instruments against other outside proteins, for example, lectins, however as a rule, it is the casein A1 protein that is at fault, not simply the milk (or the milk sugar, lactose) itself.

Besides, expectedly raised animals and their dairy items are bound with anti-infection agents and Roundup, which will send your gut mates running for the slopes. With some vital special cases that we will examine later, utilization of dairy items essentially isn't helpful for a long life and wellbeing range. On the off chance that you eat dairy items, take a note from our companions in the Blue Zones and settle on items produced using goat or sheep milk instead of dairy animals. Goats, sheep, and water wild ox were not influenced by the transformation, so their milk still contains the more beneficial casein A2 protein.

Take Away:
-   Mediterranean diets are not the answer
-   Animal Protein is not good for your gut
-   Growth hormones cause cancer
-   High metabolic rates aren't always good
-   You may be getting too much iron
-   Saturated fat is not the enemy

II: TALKIN' 'BOUT MY REGENERATION

You currently realize that a great part of the decay we ascribe to the "ordinary" maturing process is really the consequence of the crumbling of your gut divider and your microbiome, just as the Maillard response of warmth sticking together sugars and proteins inside you. Be that as it may, this decay isn't unavoidable. In the event that you treat your gut mates well, you can get more youthful as you age. The best part is that your engaged endeavors on this one zone of your body will impact fundamental changes. In the sections that pursue, we'll see how gut wellbeing impacts every individual framework in the body.

When you treat your gut amigos right, you will improve not just your gut wellbeing yet additionally your heart wellbeing, your cerebrum wellbeing, and your joint wellbeing, not to notice your weight and your skin. When we're set, you'll have a sparkling new apartment suite that is brimming with cheerful, beneficial occupants both all around.

CHAPTER 4: GET YOUNGER FROM THE INSIDE OUT

We frequently consider coronary illness as an inescapable piece of maturing. We're instructed that much the same as the remainder of us, the heart gets more fragile and more fragile as we age, and after a while you'll presumably need to go taking drugs or experience a couple of careful intercessions—possibly have your valves supplanted and your veins opened up— until, finally, your heart essentially gives out. This is ordinary, isn't that so? All things considered, when I was in medicinal school I was instructed that coronary illness is dynamic and that all we can do as doctors is attempt our best to back it off. The possibility that heart malady isn't a certainty, and that it can really be switched without medical procedure or on the other hand drug, conflicts with all that I once accepted as a heart specialist and cardiologist and everything numerous individuals and their specialists still accept. Be that as it may, what in the event that I disclosed to you that pretty much all that you've at any point been told about coronary illness is dead off-base?

Following quite a while of having a first line perspective on this organ, I've become more acquainted with the heart really well. Furthermore, what I've seen with my very own two eyes invalidates all that I was instructed about the heart as well as about our whole bodies also, our wellbeing all in all. Basically, everything returns to the safe framework— also, subsequently the gut.

I have seen confirmation of this safe assault in a significant number of my patients since I've started utilizing another blood test that has been clinically approved to anticipate your shot of showing at least a bit of kindness assault or creating angina inside the following five years. The test works by evaluating biomarkers for harm and fix occurring inside your veins. Basically, on the off chance that you have an immune system sickness or lectin affectability, this test uncovers an immune system assault on your veins that is brought in by a cytokine called interleukin 16 (IL 16).

On the off chance that your invulnerable framework is the police power of your inward condominium, you can think of interleukin 16 as a 911 administrator with the help of GPS. It alarms the cops to an accurate area. This test enables me to see that an abnormal state of interleukin 16 in a patient's blood is an indication that the cops are continually being called to the blood vessels to discover attacking Neu5Gc or lectins (or both) and end up assaulting the veins themselves. I've solicited numerous from my patients with markers characteristic of approaching heart assault issues to expel meat, pork, and sheep from their eating regimens and to restrain highlectin sustenances—and when I have retested their blood, I've discovered that their dimensions of IL 16 have fallen drastically. In certain patients, it has been decreased considerably.

This implies their odds of creating coronary illness inside the following five a long time diminished basically because of decreasing their admission of certain creature proteins and lectins. did not expand one's danger of creating coronary illness. Later examinations have demonstrated that there is no immediate association between cholesterol admission and coronary illness. The renowned China Study, which took a gander at the wellbeing and dietary propensities for individuals in sixty-five country Chinese people group thinking back to the 1990s, demonstrated that neither cholesterol utilization nor high blood dimensions of cholesterol were related with cardiovascular infection

It's not simply the heart; your gut pals control the majority of your inner organs and limits. For instance, the vast majority trust that liquor causes cirrhosis of the liver, yet in certainty you can wash the liver in liquor throughout the day and it will never create cirrhosis. What liquor in abundance causes is a broken gut by specifically harming the gut divider, which thus permits awful bugs and LPSs to enter the entryway vein, which conveys them specifically to the liver. The cops, called Kupffer cells (no, there won't be a test later), are simply hanging tight for these troublemakers to touch base in the entryway sets of three in the liver, and the fight follows. When I see raised liver chemical dimensions in a patient's blood work, I realize it is an indication of the liver fighters that have passed on or been harmed in fight. Likewise, the scar tissue that means cirrhosis is extremely an end-arrange indication of this irritation. Thus, stout men with greasy liver malady have raised dimensions of zonulin in their blood. Remember, zonulin breaks the intersections between the cells lining your gut. So greasy liver ailment is an aftereffect of a ruptured gut divider permitting intruders access into your body. New research demonstrates a much more grounded association between greasy liver ailment and the gut biome. Explicit terrible bugs increment vulnerability to greasy liver infection by animating irritation, making you bound to create cirrhosis and even liver disease, while the correct populace of gut pals can shield you from aggravation and diminish the seriousness of infection

CHAPTER 5: DANCE YOUR WAY INTO OLD AGE

For quite a long time, we trusted that joint inflammation was caused just by "mileage": the more seasoned you get, the more you utilize your joints, and in the end they simply get worn out. Be that as it may, your joints don't accompany an "utilization by" date. The latest research affirms that joint inflammation is caused not by abuse but instead by terrible bugs in the gut making aggravation. It's that aggravation that "wears and tears" your joints, not maturing itself. For example, when mice with joint pain are given enhancements of advantageous microbes, their fundamental irritation diminishes and the breakdown in ligament in their poor joint mouse knees backs off.

It's in reality extremely basic: the blend of awful bugs and a defective gut discharges lectins and LPSs into your body. Lectins tie onto the sugar particles on your joint surfaces called scialic corrosive and act like chips, inciting an insusceptible assault and irritation that prompts joint pain (and basically every other issue that we partner with maturing). Picture the red swollen region under your skin when you get a fragment; presently envision that going on inside your joints. Get the image? Those LPSs advance into your joints also and affect the same reaction.

Remember, your cops see LPSs as genuine microscopic organisms and assault. Incredibly, when we utilize a needle to draw liquid from a ligament joint, we find LPSs in the liquid! So does the mileage hypothesis identify with what's truly occurring? In a weird way, it does. Hold on for me while I get a little science geeky here. The ligament that lines your joints is always being revamped by gatherings of cells called chondrocytes and chondroblasts. (You have comparative cells that do this for your bones.) During the war in your joints, ligament is wrecked and regrown, be that as it may, this happens unevenly, bringing about strict pinnacles and valleys of ligament. The result is a sandpaper-like coating of your joints. No big surprise the specialist lets you know that your joint is "bone on bone."

Take Away:
- Not all wear and tear is due to age
- What you eat can attack your joints
- If your gut is in order then your arthritis will be better.

CHAPTER 6: REMEMBER YOUR OLD AGE

There is currently such a great amount of proof of the immediate association between gut organisms what's more, the mind that a large number of my associates have started alluding to the gut as the "second mind." I dissent—not with the immediate connection between the two but rather

Or maybe with the gut being consigned to second place. The gut really controls the mind in your mind, which you should need to begin considering as your second cerebrum. You definitely realize that your gut pals send hormonal signs or content messages to their sisters, your mitochondria, incorporating the ones in your mind.

These instant messages travel "remotely" by means of your circulatory system and lymph framework. However, your gut has another old-school method for sending messages to the "second mind" in your mind. The gut and cerebrum convey through the vagus nerve, which is the longest nerve of the autonomic sensory system and is proportional to the landline or link framework in your home. The vagus nerve controls the greater part of your autonomic (oblivious) real capacities, for example, pulse, respiratory rate, processing, etc. The vagus nerve keeps running between the gut and the cerebrum, winding around the different organs in your body en route.

When one piece of your body needs to speak with another, it makes a call along this landline to send the message. For a long time, we trusted that the vagus nerve existed for the mind (the one in your mind) to speak with what's more, offer requests to the remainder of the body, including the gut. That was what I was educated in medicinal school and accepted for quite a bit of my vocation. In any case, we currently know that it is quite other path around: for each nerve fiber driving from the cerebrum in your mind to your heart, lungs, and your gut, there are nine nerve strands prompting the mind from the last mentioned. There is along these lines nine fold the amount correspondence going from the gut to the cerebrum than there is going in the inverse heading. To say it just: your gut amigos are the ones making the calls. Not just that, yet there are in reality more neurons covering your gut to get and translate these messages than there are in your whole spinal cord.

Take Away:

- Your gut and your brain are connected
- What you eat affects your memory
- Everything in your body is connected

CHAPTER 7: LOOK YOUNGER AS YOU AGE

A few people may feel that being put resources into your appearance as you age is vain, however I deviate—all things considered, the manner in which an individual looks influences his or her selfesteem and in this way his or her psychological prosperity, which is a gigantic indicator of wellbeing results. Also, with 80 percent of the populace picking up a normal of twenty-three pounds or more since the 1980s and putting themselves at a higher danger of the considerable number of illnesses we have referenced up until this point, weight is substantially more than basically a restorative issue.

However, another motivation to concentrate on the outer is that what you see outwardly of your body is an immediate impression of the situation inside. So in the event that you've been putting on weight throughout the years and notice your skin getting more slender, all the more profoundly wrinkled, or stained over the long haul, you can make certain that something is spoiled in your center. Also, albeit some shallow changes are inescapable, it is altogether conceivable to keep up delicate, supple skin, turn around the harm that is now been done, get thinner, and show signs of improvement shape as you age.

You read before about the risks of hormone disruptors. Notwithstanding advancing early development and pubescence, these disruptors cause grown-ups to keep on put on weight as they age. This is one of the main sources of the heftiness pestilence in any case, one that couple of doctors are distinguishing in their patients who battle with their weight.

The principle hormone these synthetics upset is estrogen, which we ordinarily partner with ladies yet is really present (in changing sums) in both genders. In ladies of childbearing age, estrogen's principle work is to advise the phones to store fat to get ready for an up and coming pregnancy. This was critical back when we lived in a yearly cycle of development and relapse. Amid the development cycle, a lady would put on weight so she (and her child) could live off that put away fat amid the less fatty occasions to come. Actually, that is the reason slender female competitors in some cases try not to bleed. Their interior fat stockpiling counter doesn't think there are enough fat stores to sustain an infant and won't hazard squandering a valuable egg.

However at this point we live in a 365-day development cycle, and there is honestly no need for ladies to store fat early whether they are intending to turn into pregnant or not. Sustenance is constantly accessible for both mother and child. Be that as it may, when poisons in our condition impersonate estrogen in the body of a man or a lady, our cells get the message to store fat paying little mind to regardless of whether we are even organically equipped for getting to be pregnant. This is the reason a few young ladies are beginning adolescence at eight years old and huge numbers of my male patients previously come to me with "man boobs" and a gigantic gut that resembles a pregnancy paunch.

The possibility that minute measures of these estrogen-copying mixes could cause inconvenience has been disparaged even by those at the EPA and the FDA, whose work it is (or, tragically, was) to shield the clueless buyer from such things. Be that as it may, the aggregate impact of the moment measures of estrogen-like mixes we normally ingest from our condition is more dominant than the hormone itself would be. Rather than connecting to an estrogen receptor on a fat cell, conveying their message, and after that leaving the manner in which the ordinary estrogen hormone does, estrogen-like mixes join to the receptor and never leave, keeping the fat cell for all time changed on to continue putting away fat. This further disturbs ordinary cell informing. On account of the impacts of these mixes, men, ladies, young men, what's more, young ladies are continually putting away fat for a nonexistent forthcoming pregnancy!

Take Away:

- Your skin reflects what is going on in the inside
- Your weight could be caused by the hormones in your food
- How you eat is as important as what you eat

III: THE LONGEVITY PARADOX PROGRAM

There is truly an actual existence and-passing battle always being pursued between the heroes in your holobiome, which are committed to keeping you youthful until the day you (and they) pass on, and the miscreants, which urgently need to take over and destroy you. So the inquiry is this: Which are you going to feed and feed, and which would you say you will starve out? This is a factor in maturing that is totally inside your control. Each supper you eat and when you eat it, how what's more, the amount you work out, the items you use in the shower, the enhancements you take every day— these little decisions mean really affect your life expectancy and your wellbeing range.

For some, the clashing counsel out there—eat this, don't eat that; activity along these lines, not that way—is baffling and overpowering. A considerable lot of us simply toss our hands into the air and state, "Enough! I couldn't care less to what extent I live; simply give me what I have to feel great at the time!" Well, I'm here to reveal to you that living for the present is definitely not a triumphant procedure.

As of late I got a telephone call from a decent companion whose spouse (how about we call him Fred) has been a patient of dig for quite a long time. Fred was fit, an incredible businessperson, and the life of the gathering. Fred's significant other is a great cook, and she furthermore, Fred routinely delighted in a significant number of the nourishments I exhort against eating. For a considerable length of time, taking a gander at his lab work, I cautioned him that inconvenience was blending. In spite of his being dainty, his insulin levels were in every case high, which implied his mind was starving to death. His markers for harm to his courses were in every case high, yet he effectively breezed through the atomic pressure tests I performed on his heart. Presently Fred is in his mid seventies and all of a sudden surrendered tennis, a game he adored, in the previous a half year since he started stumbling on the court, falling, and wounding himself. All things considered, what the hell, he was getting old. Time to back off, isn't that so? In any case, over the most recent couple of months, his significant other says, he has been scanning for words what's more, just sits in his seat throughout the day, staring at the TV. A month ago, amid his office visit, I identified that "faraway look" in his eyes and alluded him to a neighborhood nervous system specialist who spends significant time in dementia. So I was, unfortunately, not amazed when his spouse called me to state that Fred had been determined to have Alzheimer's illness.

On the off chance that Fred had changed course a couple of years back, I would not be outlining for you his present result. You have gotten this far in the book since you have concluded that Fred's destiny isn't the destiny you need. Give me a chance to guarantee you, you are most certainly not alone in this adventure, and in the accompanying pages you'll adapt precisely how to settle on the best decisions for your gut mates—and in this manner for you.

CHAPTER 8: THE LONGEVITY PARADOX FOODS

There is a ton of perplexity about the distinction among probiotics and prebiotics, yet it's quite basic: though probiotics are the gut bugs themselves, prebiotics are the stringy long-chain sugars they eat. Back to our cultivating situation: probiotics are the seeds you plant in your gut garden, and prebiotics water and treat them. They do this so well since they are unpalatable by you. You can't process them, so they remain in your gut, where your gut pals can cheerfully chow down on them. Keep in mind our companions the exposed mole rodents and their consistent eating regimen of tubers, roots, and organisms? All things considered, tubers, roots, what's more, growths are superbly rich in prebiotics, which is the reason those puzzling animals have such ample and different gut amigo populaces that empower them to oppose maturing.

Notwithstanding tubers, for example, yams, jicama, and tiger nuts, rutabagas, parsnips, sweet potatoes, mushrooms, taro root (cassava), yucca, celeriac, Jerusalem artichokes (sunchokes), chicory, radicchio, artichokes, and Belgian endive are all great wellsprings of prebiotics, the last four additionally wealthy in our old companion Akkermansia's most loved nourishment: inulin. As an update, Akkermansia benefits from the defensive bodily fluid covering your gut divider and helps produce a greater amount of it. The more Akkermansia microbes you have, the more youthful you will be into ready maturity.

The kind of fat you eat is vital because most fat sources aren't impartial—they are either proinflammatory or then again mitigating. In any case, they aren't that path naturally. For example, omega-3 fats from fish oil are calming, isn't that so? All things considered, one moment. Things being what they are, the genuine calming mixes produced using DHA and EPA (two kinds of omega-3s) in fish oil are called resolvins, and these folks are the superheroes of blocking aggravation in your nerves and eyes. Be that as it may, here's the admonition: you need a tad of the dynamic fixing in headache medicine (salicylic corrosive) to get these impacts. That is the reason I suggest taking a 81-milligram enteric-covered headache medicine a couple times each week to enact that fish oil you've been gulping. Also, what about that detestable omega-6 fat arachidonic corrosive (AA), the alleged reason for irritation? All things considered, here's a mystery once more. Half of your mind's fat is the omega-3 fat DHA, while the other half is AA! What's that stuff doing up there? It's really anticipating aggravation in your mind and its memory focus, the hippocampus.

Also, in an extensive investigation of Japanese men distributed in March 2018, the men with the most abnormal amounts of AA and another omega-6 fat, linoleic corrosive (LA), had the most reduced danger of death from all causes and the least danger of cardiovascular passings! And in athletic execution preliminaries performed at Baylor University, competitors who enhanced with AA not just improved their execution contrasted and the individuals who took a fake treatment, yet (spoiler alert) a marker for irritation that I pursue, interleukin 16 (IL-16), went down essentially, not up!

The omega-3s EPA and DHA do definitely more than subdue irritation. A few contemplates demonstrate that people with the most abnormal amounts on the omega-3 record (the measure of EPA and DHA in your blood as estimated over the past two months) have the biggest cerebrum estimate and the biggest memory regions, the hippocampus, contrasted and those with the most minimal dimensions. And, as you read prior, my vegetarian patients by and large don't have a clue about that flaxseed oil, with its shortchain omega-3 fat, doesn't change over to EPA and DHA. When I first observe them, they

regularly have frightfully low omega-3 lists except if they are taking algae derived DHA. How vital is this? Consider the discoveries of an investigation from Oxford University that took a gander at the learning capacity of understudies enhanced with green growth determined DHA or a fake treatment. The individuals who took the DHA displayed improved learning and conduct, and understudies harrowed with ADHD saw an improvement in their manifestations also. Omega-3 supplements have likewise been appeared to lessen problematic conduct in sound kids. So long live fish oil, green growth determined DHA, and arachidonic corrosive! What's more, where would you be able to get both long-chain omega-3s and omega-6s? Shellfish are most likely the best decision, while egg yolk contains a lot of arachidonic corrosive alone.

Take Away:

- Omega – 3 are your friends
- Fish oils have many benefits
- You need pre and pro biotics

CHAPTER 9: THE LONGEVITY PARADOX MEAL PLAN

You currently know how imperative calorie limitation is for your wellbeing and life span. The incredible news is that you can limit calories for just five back to back outings of the month and still receive the rewards of a whole month of calorie confinement. It's hard to believe, but it's true. My companion and associate Valter Longo, leader of the Davis School of Gerontology at the University of Southern California, has demonstrated that a month to month five-day changed veggie lover quick gives you a similar life span boosting results as a month of a customary calorie-confined eating regimen does.

I unequivocally suggest that you start the Longevity Paradox program by completing five quick impersonating days straight. Not exclusively will you get similar advantages as though you had limited your calorie consumption for the entire month, yet you will drastically change the cosmetics of your gut microbes in those five days, driving out the terrible bugs and sustaining your gut pals.

- Eggs
- Soy items
- Nightshade plants (eggplant, peppers, tomatoes, potatoes)
- Corn, soy, canola, and other vegetable oils
- Meat, chicken, and all other creature items

Every other nourishment on the "Gut-Destroying Bad Bug Favorites" list

Nourishments to Include

Also, what would you be able to eat? Your gut amigos' top choices, obviously, which incorporate the following.

Vegetables

You can eat as much as you'd like of all the accompanying vegetables, either cooked or on the other hand crude. In the event that you have bad tempered gut disorder, SIBO, loose bowels, or another gut issue, limit your utilization of crude veggies and cook the remainder of the things you eat altogether. All vegetables ought to be natural and can be bought either new or solidified. Assuming crisp, they ought to be in season and developed locally with supportable cultivating rehearses, if at all conceivable.

Cruciferous vegetables: Bok choy, broccoli, Brussels grows, Swiss

chard, any shading and sort of cabbage, cauliflower, kale, mustard greens,

collard greens, rapini, kohlrabi, watercress, mizuna, arugula

Greens of numerous sorts: Belgian endive, a wide range of lettuce, spinach,

dandelion greens, chicory

Treviso, radicchio

Artichokes

Asparagus

Celery

Fennel

Radishes and other root vegetables, for example, yams, taro root, jicama,

yucca, cassava, turnips, rutabagas, horseradish

Crisp herbs: Mint, parsley, sage, basil, and cilantro, in addition to garlic what not

sorts of onions, including leeks and chives

Sea vegetables: Kelp and ocean growth, including sheets of nori

Protein

For these five days, you will go veggie lover. That implies no eggs, meat,

chicken, or dairy results of any sort. Try not to stress that you will turn into protein insufficient! Keep in mind, you are presumably eating an excessive amount of protein right presently, and your body reuses the protein that is as of now present. Taking out creature items for five days gives your body a rest from processing all that protein and enables it to turn into an eco-accommodating retreat for your gut mates! Wellsprings of plant-based protein that you can eat amid these five days (in amounts of eight ounces every day or less) incorporate yet don't need to include:

Tempeh (aged soy, without grains)

Hemp tofu and hemp seeds

Weight cooked vegetables, for example, lentils and beans

Hilary's Millet Cakes

Affirmed nuts and seeds

Keep in mind, your incredible chimp cousins and your predecessors got a lot of protein by eating leaves, and you can also.

Fats and Oils

Satisfactory vegetable fat hotspots for these five days include:

Avocado—don't hesitate to have an entire one every day

First-cool squeezed additional virgin olive oil

Olives of any sort

Nuts: Walnuts, macadamia nuts, pistachios, hazelnuts, pine nuts,

Marcona almonds, whitened almond flour

Avocado oil

Coconut oil

Macadamia nut oil

MCT oil

Perilla oil

Sesame seed oil

Walnut oil

Hemp seed oil

Flaxseed oil

Sauces and Seasonings

As a result of their sugar content (also other hurtful fixings), keep away from all monetarily arranged plate of mixed greens dressings and sauces. Rather, use as much as you like of the accompanying.

Crisp lemon juice

Vinegars

Mustard

Newly ground dark pepper

Iodized ocean salt

Your most loved herbs and flavors, less red bean stew pepper chips

Drinks

Clearly, you will evade all soft drinks (counting diet soft drink), sports drinks, lemonade, and other monetarily arranged refreshments. Rather, appreciate in any event some tap or sifted water multi day.

Take Away

- Stay away from Proteins
- Go for healthy fats
- Drink ½ your body weight in ounces

CHAPTER 10: THE LONGEVITY PARADOX LIFESTYLE PLAN

One reason calorie confinement is helpful is that it briefly stresses your phones, and a smidgen of stress is something worth being thankful for: it sends a flag to your cells that they ought to get ready for an approaching danger to your and their survival. This powers them to toughen up and executes off any cells that can't be reinforced and thusly aren't probably going to endure the invasion. It is one of the most gainful things you can do to advance your wellbeing and life span.

That is the reason the following mainstay of the Longevity Paradox program includes focusing on your cells through your eating routine as well as through your way of life decisions. As you start this adventure, it's vital to remember that the more you stress your body, the additional time you have to recuperate, or you hazard pushing yourself to an extreme and causing more damage than anything else. So getting a lot of rest furthermore, setting aside some effort to unwind or reflect are likewise basic parts of this program. Switching back and forth between times of pressure and revival is another cycle that will profit your gut mates and help you accomplish a long wellbeing length.

In light of this, I've separated the way of life program into two sections: first, the propensities that will pressure and reinforce your cells, and second, the propensities that will enable them to recuperate. Together, these basic way of life alterations will abandon you—and your gut amigos—feeling like nothing anyone's ever seen.

Exercise is a standout amongst the most ordinarily polished types of hormesis. Without fail you work out, you make little tears in your muscles. At the point when your muscles fix themselves, they become more grounded and greater. Also, as you read prior, your gut amigos likewise advantage when you practice and reimburse you by repairing their home. They particularly like it when you practice against gravity since this burdens— furthermore, consequently reinforces— a greater amount of your muscles.

In the event that you are worried that you're not fit as a fiddle and can't securely begin a weight preparing convention, have no dread. Jack LaLanne, "the Godfather of Modern Wellness," instructed me that you have to do just two basic activities to create and look after quality. Those two activities are squats (or any sort of profound knee curves) and boards or push-ups. The two activities neutralize gravity, and together they stress each real muscle assemble in the body. Anybody at any wellness level can do them, and only a little venture of time will yield significant outcomes.

My five-minute exercise plan joins these developments and three others you'll perceive for a total, balanced exercise that gives the sum of stress your muscles need to remain solid and avert squandering, or loss of muscle mass with age. You have no reason to abstain from doing this. Begin off by finishing this circuit two times every day or at whatever point you want to get up and get going, particularly on the off chance that you spend an expansive segment of your day sitting. It will give you an moment burst of vitality while reinforcing every one of the muscles—and cells—in your body.

Exercise is a standout amongst the most ordinarily rehearsed types of hormesis. Inevitably you work out, you make small tears in your muscles. At the point when your muscles fix themselves, they become more grounded and greater. Furthermore, as you read prior, your gut pals likewise advantage when you practice and reimburse you by repairing their home. They particularly like it when you practice against gravity since this burdens—what's more, in this way fortifies—a greater amount of your muscles.

On the off chance that you are worried that you're not fit as a fiddle and can't securely begin a weight preparing convention, have no dread. Jack LaLanne, "the Godfather of Modern Wellness," instructed me that you have to do just two basic activities to create and look after quality. Those two activities are squats (or any kind of profound knee twists) and boards or push-ups. The two activities neutralize gravity, and together they stress each significant muscle aggregate in the body. Anybody at any wellness level can do them, and only a little speculation of time will yield important outcomes.

My five-minute exercise plan fuses these developments and three others you'll perceive for a total, balanced exercise that gives the sum of stress your muscles need to remain solid and avoid squandering, or loss of muscle mass with age. You have no reason to abstain from doing this. Begin off by finishing this circuit two times per day or at whatever point you want to get up and get going, particularly on the off chance that you spend a substantial segment of your day sitting. It will give you an moment burst of vitality while reinforcing every one of the muscles—and cells—in your body.

Exercise is a standout amongst the most usually rehearsed types of hormesis. Unfailingly you work out, you make small tears in your muscles. At the point when your muscles fix themselves, they become more grounded and greater. Also, as you read prior, your gut amigos additionally advantage when you practice and reimburse you by repairing their home.

They particularly like it when you practice against gravity since this anxieties— what's more, in this manner reinforces—a greater amount of your muscles. In the event that you are worried that you're not fit as a fiddle and can't securely begin a weight preparing convention, have no dread. Jack LaLanne, "the Godfather of Modern Wellness," instructed me that you have to do just two basic activities to create and look after quality. Those two activities are squats (or any sort of profound knee twists) and boards or push-ups. The two activities neutralize gravity, and together they stress each significant muscle assemble in the body. Anybody at any wellness level can do them, and only a little venture of time will yield significant outcomes.

My five-minute exercise plan joins these developments and three others you'll perceive for a total, balanced exercise that gives the sum of stress your muscles need to remain solid and counteract squandering, or loss of muscle mass with age. You have no reason to abstain from doing this. Begin off by finishing this circuit two times every day or at whatever point you want to get up and get going, particularly on the off chance that you spend a vast segment of your day sitting. It will give you an moment burst of vitality while reinforcing every one of the muscles—and cells—in your body.

Take Away

- Exercise is a great stress reliever
- Heat is healing so get sweating
- Get moving to get healing

CHAPTER 11: LONGEVITY PARADOX SUPPLEMENT RECOMMENDATIONS

Numerous individuals still trust that there is an enhancement enchantment projectile—in other words, that at least one enhancements will by one way or another right their continuous dependence on the common Western eating routine, just as cause all their medical problems to mystically turn around course and mend their bodies. Additionally, on the off chance that you examine the Web, you will discover wild cases that taking one specific enhancement will make you unfading or nearly. I can guarantee you this is jabber, and I state that since I have seen this confusion in my patients' blood work far too often in the course of the most recent eighteen years. Be that as it may, on the off chance that you leave on the Life span Paradox program, huge numbers of the enhancements that pursue can and will give quantifiable advantages. I have displayed contemplates on such advantages at national and universal therapeutic meetings. Keep in mind, consistent with their name, supplements upgrade the consequences of the Longevity Paradox program—however they are not alternate ways.

A few of my associates in life span take the doctor prescribed medication metformin what's more, some in any event talk about and may furtively take the organ transplant antirejection medicate rapamycin (Sirolimus), the last for its known direct concealment of mTOR. I do not one or the other, leaning toward the regular techniques I have illustrated in this book and utilizing other common enhancements to emulate these medications' activities. A disclaimer: I possess and work my very own enhancement organization, GundryMD, yet not the slightest bit am I proposing that you have to purchase my items. I have consolidated a large number of my most loved supplements together in equations for GundryMD.com. be that as it may, I additionally share the names of different brands I like, just as the supplement dose, so you can discover whatever works best for you and your financial plan, either on the web or in your nearby wellbeing nourishment store.

I used to tell my patients that supplements made costly pee. That was before I began estimating the impacts of nutrients, minerals, and plant mixes, for example, polyphenols, flavonoids, and different phytonutrients on my patients' irritation biomarkers. I can now dependably observe when patients have changed their enhancement routine or even changed brands, in view of these tests.

Our seeker gatherer progenitors devoured in excess of 250 unique plants every year on a pivoting, regular premise. Those plants' foundations dug profound into six feet of natural topsoil soil, which overflowed with microbes and parasites to make an astounding mix of minerals and phytochemicals inside the plants' tubers, leaves, blossoms, and natural products. The meat and fat from the creatures that our progenitors murdered and ate additionally contained those phytochemicals, in light of the fact that the creatures they ate likewise ate those plants.

Suppose that you eat natural sustenance, you eat regularly, you visit your neighborhood ranchers' market, you expend wild-got fish, you limit your utilization of fed chicken and eggs, you limit your utilization of grass-bolstered meats, what's more, you sprinkle matured cheeses from A2 bovines, just as from sheep and goats, on your sustenance. You eat weight cooked lentils; you toss mushrooms on everything. You skip dinners, you have a mentally condition night week by week. Isn't that enough?

As the lab tests on a considerable lot of my patients who are dependable natural eaters appear, getting the majority of the supplements you need just is impossible in our general public without taking enhancements. Lamentably (or maybe luckily), you don't live in Okinawa during the 1940s, on Kitava, or on a remote island off the bank Greece; you get my float. So here are a couple of the enhancements that I prescribe considering. The first two—nutrient D3 and the B nutrients—are fundamental for everybody.

Take Away

- Natural Supplements can help your gut
- Chemicals are not always the answer
- You can live off all natural foods

CHAPTER 12: LONGEVITY PARADOX RECIPES

Life span Leek Soup

The leeks in this soup are a brilliant life span nourishment with heaps of polyphenols. Far superior, it is flawless to eat amid your five-day "quick." It has a splendid lemony flavor with a wealth from the nutmeg that will keep you warm throughout the day.

Serves 4 to 6

Ingredients

2 tablespoons additional virgin olive oil
1 pound leeks, cleaned and hacked
2 stalks celery, diced
3 cloves garlic, minced
1 tablespoon hacked new thyme
juice of 1 lemon
1 extensive head cauliflower, cut into 2-inch florets
1/2 teaspoon crisp nutmeg
1 teaspoon fine ocean salt, or more to taste
2 teaspoons coarse dark pepper
2 quarts vegetable stock
1 straight leaf

Directions

Finely cleaved chives for enhancement
In a substantial soup pot, heat the olive oil over medium-high warmth. Include the leeks, celery, garlic, thyme, lemon pizzazz, and cauliflower alongside the nutmeg, salt, furthermore, pepper, and sauté over medium warmth, mixing normally until the leeks start to shrink.

Include the stock and the inlet leaf and cook, secured, for 25 to 35 minutes, until the cauliflower is delicate. Mix utilizing a stick blender, or move into a normal blender and mix until smooth (work in bunches so as not to stuff the blender).

Once pureed, come back to the warmth and cook for an extra 10 to 15 minutes.

Taste, and alter flavoring as required. Serve embellished with slashed chives.

Lentil Miso Soup with Shiitake Mushrooms

At the point when the climate's crisp, there's not at all like a rich, hearty bean soup — and this one is loaded with polyamines and other antiaging mixes, what's sans more of lectins!

Serves 4

Ingredients

2 tablespoons additional virgin olive oil
1 extensive shallot, finely slashed
3 cloves garlic, minced
1 container meagerly cut crisp shiitake mushrooms
11/2 tablespoons new thyme, minced
1 tablespoon new rosemary, minced
3 tablespoons red miso glue
6 containers Parmesan "Bone" Broth or mushroom juices
11/2 containers weight cooked lentils (Eden brand canned lentils alright)
1 glass cut kale, stems evacuated
Coconut aminos, to taste

Directions

In an expansive soup pot, heat the olive oil over medium-high warmth. Include the shallot also, garlic and cook, blending much of the time, until the shallot is delicate and the garlic is fragrant, around 3 minutes.

Decrease the warmth to medium and include the mushrooms, thyme, and rosemary. Cook an extra 3 to 4 minutes, mixing regularly, until the mushrooms are delicate.

Include the miso glue and cook, mixing always, until the glue is
fused into the vegetable blend.

Include the soup and lentils and cook for 20 to 30 minutes, secured.

Include the kale and cook, revealed, an extra 20 minutes, until the kale is shriveled and the soup is marginally thickened.

Include the coconut aminos a tad at any given moment, tasting until you like the flavor, at that point serve.

Rich Cauliflower Parmesan Soup

This soup is best made with the Parmesan "Bone" Broth — it truly features the kinds of the cauliflower. On the off chance that you cherish a leek and potato soup or chowder, odds are this soup will be definitely fit for your abilities. Also, it's loaded with cruciferous cauliflower and cerebrum boosting olive oil.

Serves 6

Ingredients

3 tablespoons additional virgin olive oil
1 sweet onion, minced
2 stalks celery, diced
3 cloves garlic, minced
2 extensive heads cauliflower, cut into 2-inch florets
1/2 teaspoon new ground nutmeg
1 teaspoon fine ocean salt, or to taste
2 teaspoons coarse dark pepper
1 tablespoon white miso glue
7 containers mushroom stock or Parmesan "Bone" Broth
2 containers coconut milk
1/4 container ground Parmesan cheddar or healthful yeast
1 sound leaf

Directions

Finely hacked chives or thyme for embellishment In an extensive soup pot, heat the olive oil over medium-high warmth. Include the onion, celery, garlic, and cauliflower, alongside the nutmeg, salt, and pepper, and sauté over medium warmth, mixing consistently, until the leeks start to shrivel.

Include the miso glue and cook, mixing, until the glue is fused. Include the stock, coconut milk, Parmesan, and inlet leaf and cook, secured, for 35 to 45 minutes, until the cauliflower is delicate. Mix utilizing a stick blender, or move into a normal blender and mix until smooth (work in bunches so as not to overload the blender).

Once pureed, come back to the warmth and cook an extra 10 to 15 minutes. In the event that it is excessively thick, dainty with a little water. Taste and modify the flavoring as required. Serve decorated with slashed herbs and extra ground Parmesan.

Severe Green Salad with Walnut Blue Cheese Dressing

As I generally state, all the more severe, all the more better. Your most loved gut pal, Akkermansia, cherishes these greens! In any case, have no dread in case you're not a fan of very harsh flavors and still need to profit by expending severe nourishments. The fat in this plate of mixed greens dressing and the sweetness of the cranberries balance out the sharpness from the veggies wonderfully.

Serves 2

Ingredients

For the dressing:
1/4 container disintegrated matured blue cheddar, ideally French or Italian
1/4 container red wine vinegar
1/4 container additional virgin olive oil
1/2 container toasted walnuts
Juice of 1/2 lemon

For the plate of mixed greens:
2 mugs destroyed kale
1 container destroyed or hacked endive or radicchio
1/4 container minced new dill (I concede I'd overlook this, however my significant other cherishes it)
1/4 container minced crisp parsley
1 avocado, cut into pieces
1/4 container unsweetened dried cranberries

Directions

MAKE THE DRESSING:

Combine all the dressing fixings in a blender or in a sustenance processor fitted with a S sharp edge. Heartbeat until smooth, diminishing with water as required (it ought to be the consistency of farm or blue cheddar dressing).

MAKE THE SALAD:
Combine the kale, endive, dill, and parsley in an expansive bowl. Include a large portion of the dressing and hurl until the greens are very much covered. Top the plate of mixed greens with avocado and cranberries, and present with the remaining dressing.

Sweet Potato and Coconut Pudding

This treat is propelled by an Asian pastry including taro, yet sweet potatoes are frequently less demanding to discover in your market and have loads of safe starch in their very own right. It's not the best sweet, however the flavors are mind blowing: coconut, vanilla, and cinnamon play perfectly together, making it feel wanton and light in the meantime.

Serves 4

Ingredients

1 container custard pearls
2 containers coconut milk
1 container unsweetened destroyed coconut
1/4 teaspoon cinnamon
1 teaspoon vanilla concentrate
1/4 container erythritol powder
2 containers stripped, diced sweet potatoes or taro root

Directions

In a little pot, heat some water to the point of boiling. Include the custard pearls also, bubble for 10 minutes, at that point expel from the warmth and spread. Let rest for 20 minutes.

While the custard is cooking, heat the coconut milk, destroyed coconut, cinnamon, vanilla, and erythritol powder over medium warmth, blending at times. Include the sweet potatoes and keep on cooking until delicate, 15 to 20 minutes contingent upon how little you've cut them.

At the point when the sweet potatoes are delicate, strain the water off the custard pearls and add them to the coconut blend. Cook for an extra 2 minutes. Serve warm, or exchange to the cooler and serve chilled for a custard like surface.

Take Away:

- Eating Healthy Should be delicious
- If you don't make delicious, you won't want to eat it
- Eating right should leave you full and happy
- If you feel good about what you eat, your gut will be happy too.

Afterword

The oddity of life span comes down to this: No one's getting out alive. In any case you can kick the bucket youthful at a ready maturity by collecting the correct group. Or on the other hand, maybe all the more precisely, by amassing a town of trillions of occupants who need just a single thing, and that is to save their delightful home. Your group ought to likewise incorporate a dedicated accumulation of relatives, companions, and creatures who can furnish you with enthusiastic and social help and motivate you to remain dynamic consistently.

Be that as it may, we should not overlook the significance of your frame of mind on your personal satisfaction. One of the qualities I've seen in huge numbers of the "excessively old" individuals I've had the delight of knowing is a viewpoint I like to call skeptical good faith. It's exemplified by the life-upgrading capacity to shrug your shoulders at the inescapable terrible things that occur and commend the numerous beneficial things. For instance, I'll abandon you to mull over Ruby, who is turning 102 as I compose this. I've known Ruby for no less than ten years. When I met her, this modest lady had hands and feet that were so contorted and disfigured by rheumatoid joint inflammation that my first inquiry to her was, didn't it hurt appallingly to walk? Her reaction was what I have generally expected from my extraordinary instructors: "Of course it harms, yet I can't take care of business, so why give it any consideration?" She shrugged. What's more, grinned. All the while. What's more, in her eyes I identified the extraordinary shimmer of life that gave a false representation of her actual age. In her nineties, she showed seat yoga! She had a nearby system of companions. I started to anticipate each visit with Ruby, not on the grounds that she was such a delight to be near yet additionally in light of the fact that I generally taken in something from her. After quite a long time after year I would recommend that we attempt a couple of dietary changes to help with her rheumatoid joint inflammation, yet she simply wasn't intrigued. Not long after her 100th birthday she found a bump in her bosom that was destructive and must be expelled. When we met after her medical procedure, I asked her what her arrangements were currently that she was 100 and had malignant growth. Once more, her answer didn't astound me. She needed to live to see her extraordinary grandkids move on from secondary school and wouldn't give a seemingly insignificant detail a chance to like malignant growth remain in her direction. I inquired as to whether maybe now was an ideal opportunity to attempt the dietary changes I had been recommending, and she at long last stated, "Beyond any doubt, Doc, we out it an attempt."

At the point when Ruby strolled in the entryway for her 101st birthday visit, I was right away struck by the presence of her hands. The frightfully distorted knuckles were presently significantly littler, and her fingers and toes were discernibly straighter. A brisk look at her fresh recruits work results demonstrated to me that her biomarkers for dynamic rheumatoid joint pain, RF and Anti-CCP3, which were typically very raised, were presently ordinary. As in negative. I energetically disclosed to her that her eating endeavors had satisfied, demonstrating her the blood results and indicating her loose hands. She stated, "Truly, I've seen my hands, yet I have an unresolved issue with you." With that she turned her hands and fingers toward the floor, and six rings tumbled off her fingers, banging onto the tile. "I must get my rings resized!" The ideal cynical self assured person in real life.

Ruby's deaging is occurring directly before my eyes; presently, at 102, she just keeps getting more youthful. Also, this is my desire for you. Through a mix of nourishment, way of life decisions, a strong network, and an outlook that looks for the positive while tolerating the negative with silliness and quietude, we can all appreciate a full, dynamic life for the same number of years as we live on this planet.

Obviously, Ruby's a great opportunity to move forward will in the long run come, similarly as my time what's more, yours will. However, until it does, I for one intend to support that crucial flash that keeps her birthday candles lit quite a long time after year. Or on the other hand as Jason Mraz would state, "May the best of your todays be the most noticeably bad of your tomorrows." Die youthful, dear peruser, at a ready seniority!

Take Away
- You can eat for your health
- The key to a long, happy life is knowing how food affects you
- It is easy to be healthy